How to Choose a Baby Formula

Garry Wainscott, M.Hlth.Sci.(Hum.Nutr.)

DISCLAIMER

The material in this publication is of the nature of general comment only and does not represent medical or professional advice. It is not intended to provide specific guidance for particular circumstances and it should not be relied upon as the basis for any decision to take action or not take action on any matter which it covers. Readers should obtain professional advice where appropriate, before making any such decision. To the maximum extent permitted by law, the author disclaims all responsibility and liability to any person, arising directly or indirectly from any person taking or not taking action based upon the information in this publication.

How to Choose a Baby Formula
© 2012, Garry Wainscott
Perth, Western Australia

Cover: Photograph by courtesy of Philips Electronics Australia

ISBN: 1475122691
ISBN 13: 9781475122695

CONTENTS

About the Author

Garry Wainscott, born in New Zealand, is a pharmacist by trade and dispensed both human and veterinary treatments prior to moving into the pharmaceutical industry. After eight years with the first company he worked for, he became a key manager with a major US-based international company involved both in pharmaceuticals and in nutrition products. Eventually Garry was promoted to a general management position.

After nine years with that company in New Zealand, he transferred to Asian postings, living and working in Indonesia, Singapore, and Thailand in key marketing roles and general management. He spent twenty-six years managing operations both in Southeast Asia and in South Asia before retiring to start his own business, TeknoLink Nutrition, based in Perth, Western Australia.

Garry's involvement with infant nutrition began in 1967 when he lobbied the dairy industry and the Department of Agriculture in New Zealand to be permitted to remove the saturated fats from cow milk and replace them with vegetable oils to initiate infant formula manufacturing in that country. Working with three regional paediatric groups in Sri Lanka and organising analytical services in the Nutrition Department, University of Otago, Dunedin, New Zealand, he enabled the first Sri Lankan breast milk studies in the 1990s.

Whilst domiciled in Singapore, Garry held multi-year tenures as president of the Singapore Association of Pharmaceutical Industries (SAPI) and chairman of the Advertising Standards Authority of Singapore (ASAS). In 1983 he founded the Singapore Nutrition and Dietetics Association (SNDA).

From 2003 to 2006, Garry lectured on various infant nutrition topics to paediatricians at various venues in Malaysia, Indonesia, Sri Lanka, Philippines, China, Hong Kong, and Taiwan. He was a guest speaker at the 2005 Obstetrics & Gynaecology of Singapore Congress and a guest speaker at the 2006 Obstetrical & Gynaecology Society of Malaysia Congress

Garry graduated from Deakin University, Australia:
>Graduate Diploma in Human Nutrition
>Master of Health Science (Human Nutrition).

Acknowledgments

Special thanks go to Lily Withers, my joint venture partner, for her insights that relate to the potential readers of this book. This book was written for "mums-to-be", new mums, and mums faced with the challenges of breast-feeding, as well as for those who are simply interested in seeking up-to-date information on baby formulas.

I also extend special thanks to the small group of senior pædiatricians and neonatologists in Singapore who several years ago invited me to a special round table discussion evening for them to learn in greater depth the latest developments in baby formulas. That discussion encouraged me to pursue further the goal of making those research conclusions more widely known.

Prelude

If you expect to find a convenient list of brand-named products, ranked in order of superior nutritional benefit or baby development benefit, you will not find it in these pages.

Instead you will find explanations of some of the key attributes present in baby formulas, which can help you better consider which formula may be most suitable for your baby. Once you gain a better understanding of the baby formulas you may be considering, your choice is ultimately up to you. After all, such a choice is important, as Baby gets only one start in Life. Your personal choice also may take into account both your own baby's requirements and your own situation, including relative cost between baby formulas.

There are many manufacturers of baby formulas, some renowned, and some not so well known. Often manufacturers offer various brands, some priced at a lower level, with the main objective of keeping a baby alive and reasonably healthy. These companies' other brands may contain expensive ingredients designed to provide better brain and eye development, help a baby resist infection, or make other claims, and therefore they will charge more for these formulas

Some manufacturers brand their products differently from country to country. Not all baby formulas are available in all countries due to marketing limits, local regulations, insufficient opportunity for viable profitability, and lack of practical distribution avenues.

For these reasons this book is intended to provide you with the knowledge and understanding to better assess the baby formulas that are available where you live.

Can a Baby Formula Help My Baby Have a Good Start in Life?

It is well accepted that the best possible start in Life a baby can have, is access to its own mother's breast milk. For this reason modern-day baby formulas are based on average breast milk nutrient values and levels, which are regarded as "The Gold Standard".

It is also understood that many mothers experience either great difficulty in breast feeding or, for a variety of reasons, prefer not to breast feed or cease exclusive breast feeding after a period of time. These mothers should feel no "guilt" in so doing. A study performed by two health boards in Scotland and published in 2012 in the *British Medical Journal* resulted in a suggestion that breastfeeding advice should be realistic, not idealistic. The study concluded that *"Adopting idealistic global policy goals like exclusive breast feeding until 6 months as individual goals for women is unhelpful. More achievable incremental goals are recommended."*

"Exclusive breast feeding" is defined as providing a baby, from birth, with no other substance (not even water) apart from breast milk and prescribed medicines. Rather than being nutritionally based, guidelines from the World Health Organisation (WHO) that recommend exclusive breast-feeding are probably more directed at preventing illness, gastroenteritis, and infection during early babyhood in those environments where sanitation and hygiene during preparation of baby formula and bottles and utensils may be poor. In developed countries where good sanitation and hygiene practices are the norm, exclusive breast-feeding may not be so critical.

An initial period of breast feeding can provide a baby with the "humoral" aspects of some immunoglobulins and maternal cells. If a baby does not receive the initial flow of breast milk, however, how much is that baby's health and wellbeing compromised? My own mother was unable to breast feed me from birth, and I barely survived on a small number of concoctions that were available in those days before baby formulas became available. As a champion middle-distance runner and cross-country runner, with a successful management career and "mature student" achievements, as well as decades of good health, I have never considered myself at a disadvantage to those who were breast fed as babies.

In reality, it is also acknowledged that breast milk is anything but "standard" in nature. Composition varies significantly during the duration of each feed, composition also can differ from feed to feed, and the fats in a mother's breast milk reflect to some extent the day-to-day consumption of fats in her diet. In addition the provision of some nutrients to the baby can be diminished if the mother has a particular nutrient deficiency or deficiencies.

At about four months of age, Baby's iron needs greatly increase, and breast milk can no longer meet these demands for iron. With the rapid growth in Baby's size during this period, breast milk does not provide sufficient vitamin D, and by six months of age, Baby's protein needs are no longer met if breast milk is the sole source of nutrition. This is the reason exclusive breast-feeding is recommended only up to six months of age. In Myanmar (also known as Burma), over-zealous officials promoted exclusive breast-feeding until at least eight months of age. The result? Whereas there was very little malnutrition at six months of age, by twelve months of age 75 percent of babies in Myanmar showed symptoms of malnutrition.

Only one hundred to 120 years ago, babies who were unable to receive their own mothers' breast milk had to rely on "wet nurses" (other mothers who were still lactating) for nourishment. With a shortage of wet nurses, there was a high death rate among those babies who did not have access to the services of a wet nurse. During the latter part of the first half of the twentieth century, some rather basic baby formulas became available, which increased the survival rates in babies who were unable to receive their own mothers' breast milk.

These baby formulas also led to the ability of scientists to appreciate the importance of various component nutrients of breast milk in relation to the growth and development of babies. This ability comes from the standardisation of a formula, then the ability to increase or lower the amount of specific nutrients, for use in clinical evaluation.

In the early 1950s, scientific acknowledgment that babies poorly absorbed the saturated fats present in cow milk led to formulations based on non-fat cow milk with added vegetable oils as the fat source. These were the first of the so-called "humanised" baby formulas. There are two broad categories of protein in milk, the casein fraction and the whey fraction. Cow milk protein is very predominant in the casein fraction (about 80 percent), whereas breast milk is more predominantly whey protein (about 60 percent) than casein protein (approximately 40 percent). Developments in the dairy industry in the 1970s enabled manufacturers to provide ultra-filtrated whey protein concentrate (to reduce the heavy load of minerals in cow milk), which permitted baby formulas to better imitate the whey-to-protein ratios of breast milk. This advance marked yet another milestone in baby formula development.

Since then there have been many more "milestones" in baby formula formulation, and today the marketplace offers many highly sophisticated baby formulas that rightly can claim to be able to give your baby a good start in Life.

What Types of Baby Formula are Available?

For our discussion, the term "babies" is interchangeable with "infants," who, by definition, are zero to twelve months old. For babies who do not have special needs, two types of baby formulas are available.

Stage 1 Formula (also known as "starter formula").

Stage 1 formula is designed to match as closely as scientifically possible with breast milk in all key nutrient parameters. It is intended for use when breast-feeding is not possible or available during the first six months of a baby's life. A mother also may use Stage 1 formula if she needs to supplement breast-feeding during this period.

Stage 2 Formula (also known as "follow-on formula").

Stage 2 formula is designed to provide adequate amounts of key nutrients that may not be present in adequate amounts in the semisolid and solid weaning foods that Baby will be receiving in the second six months of babyhood. Stage 2 formula is therefore not quite as rigidly equated to breast milk.

For convenience both in marketing and in comprehension by mothers, there is a suggestion that at around six months of age, an infant who receives Stage 1 baby formula should be switched to Stage 2 baby formula. There is, however, no hard and fast rule to this. Babies are individuals, and their growth rates and development may decide the timing of a switch from Stage 1 to Stage 2 formula. In the case of my granddaughters, breast-feeding was supplemented with Stage 1 baby formula from four months of age. At eight months of age, during diminishing breast-feeding, their diet was supplemented with Stage 2 formula. When they were thirteen months old, breast-feeding ceased, and they continued to receive Stage 2 formula until around two years of age. This raises another issue.

Well-meaning advisors often instil a fear into some mothers that babies should not be introduced to nurser (bottle) feeding (either for water or supplementary feeding). They suggest that once babies drink from a nurser they will no longer accept breast-feeding. Experience over many years has convinced me that this is an erroneous assumption. Many mothers feed their babies by nursers during the day then settle their babies in the evening with breast-feeding in the hope of helping their babies achieve better nightly sleep patterns. Their babies appear to experience no problems in switching from breast to bottle and back to breast again.

At about four months of age, Baby begins to develop the muscular coordination and ability to shift food from the front of the mouth to the rear of the mouth in preparation for swallowing.

Encouragement for development of the swallowing reflex (the ability to automatically shut off the airways whenever swallowing takes place in order to avoid choking) and the fact that Baby is beginning to outgrow the ability of either breast milk or baby formula to meet all of his/her daily nutrient needs prompt the introduction of small increments of semisolid foods then, later, more solid forms of food.

Babies tend to take in quantities of milk or formula that meet their daily energy requirements; this means they tend to drink as many calories as they need. The daily intake from breast milk increases progressively from birth until it reaches the limit of the mother's daily ability to produce breast milk. Generally this is approximately 750 ml per day, although for some population groups (e.g., Australians) average daily intake from breast milk is calculated at 850 ml. In cases of multiple births, daily breast milk volumes of one litre are not uncommon. The daily volume of baby formula available does not have these constraints, and by about three months of age it is not uncommon for a baby to receive one litre of baby formula per day. Therefore, studies that show that formula-fed babies grow in both weight and length at a faster rate than breast-fed babies do not show that baby formula is "better" than breast milk but reflect instead a greater daily energy and protein intake in formula-fed babies.

Some babies have special formula needs. For example, premature babies, babies with family histories of allergies, and babies with metabolic disorders require appropriately modified formulas. The choice of baby formula in these circumstances is more a matter of recommendation by a paediatric specialist than a choice on the part of the mother.

Cow Milk is for Calves

Whole cow milk should *not* be fed to babies. The milk of every mammalian species is different and appropriately tailored to the unique needs of the individual species. The calf of a cow, very soon after birth, unsteadily gets to its feet and follows its mother to begin suckling from her udder.

A calf's nutrient requirements are very different to those of a human infant, who, following birth, is helplessly dependent upon its mother to cradle and nurse it and does not become ambulatory until one year of age or soon thereafter.

In other words the human infant is born at a far earlier stage of development relative to that of a calf. This variation in at-birth development levels requires that the human infant ingest various nutrients at levels very different to what the calves of cows require. This is why quality infant formulas were created.

Undiluted whole cow milk has a protein level that is considered too high for the feeding of infants, and the American Academy of Pediatrics (AAP) strongly recommends that whole cow milk should *not* be fed to babies during their first twelve months of life. Undiluted whole cow milk also has been well documented as a cause of intestinal blood loss in infants. The presence of blood in the stools is a common finding among infants with iron deficiency anaemia. Approximately one-half of such babies experience blood in their stools, and blood loss may average approximately 1.5 ml per day. The feeding of undiluted cow milk leads to increased blood loss in the intestinal-tract in a large proportion of normal babies, and the amount of iron lost in this blood is nutritionally important.

Saturated fatty acids in cow milk account for 63 percent of its total fat content. In comparison, saturated fatty acids account for only 43 percent of the total fat in breast milk. When infants receive homogenized and pasteurized fresh cow milk as their sole source of energy, fat excretions are generally more than 20 percent and often more than 30 percent of intake. Quality infant formulas endeavour to mimic the fatty acid profile of human breast milk as closely as possible by using plant-based fats (vegetable oils) rather than cow milk fats.

Cow milk has a low concentration of iron—only about 0.1 – 0.2 mg per litre. Furthermore, iron absorption studies in infants demonstrate that the absorption of this iron is low. Cow milk is qualitatively a very poor supplier of iron for babies. It also contains very low levels of vitamin A, and its vitamin D levels are almost nonexistent. Vitamin A deficiency is a public health problem in more than 50 percent of countries, especially in Africa and Southeast Asia, according to the World Health Organisation.

Vitamin A deficiency is a cause of blindness in up to five hundred thousand children each year. Vitamin A deficiency is most prevalent in Asia, especially in Indonesia, India, Bangladesh, and the Philippines, as well as in parts of Africa. Recently the importance of dietary vitamin D intake has become better appreciated. As a result, recommended intake levels have been increased to more than those formerly advocated. In 2008 the American Academy of Pediatrics called for a doubling of recommended vitamin D intake levels and subsequently the National Academy of Science's Institute of Medicine (IOM) increased the Recommended Dietary Allowances for babies up to 12 months of age from 200 iu per day to 400 iu per day. Cow milk is exceptionally low in vitamin D, and even human milk vitamin D levels are considered to be inadequate for developing infants. A recent study found that in the US states with highest exclusive breastfeeding rates the incidence of autism also was highest (Vitamin D and Autism: Critical Review, Re Dev Disabil 2012 33(5):1541-1550). Unless the mother takes 5.000 IU of vitamin D per day and has vitamin D level greater than 40 ng/ml, her breast milk contains little vitamin D (Vitamin D Council, May 2, 2012).

The Committee on Nutrition of the American Academy of Pediatrics categorically states: *"The only acceptable alternative to breast milk is iron-fortified infant formula. Appropriate solid foods should be added between the ages of 4 and 6 months."*

Those Pretty Labels

When selecting a baby formula, a mother is often faced with label "claims" that can be confusing and sometimes misleading. A typical example is the claim that a "unique" combination of nutrients will "help support" a baby's immune system. Sounds impressive? Especially when a brand encloses the claim within a "shield" (what else?) emblazoned with the trademarked name "Immunocare".

In the majority of such baby formula "claims" a closer inspection of such a "unique" blend usually reveals a mixture of individual nutrients that, independently, are suggested in textbooks to be somehow involved in the immune process of the body. When these nutrients are blended into the baby formula, the manufacturer then claims they "nutritionally support the developing immune system". Note: A manufacturer will not make a direct claim that your baby is likely to be able to resist infections as a result of taking a particular baby formula. The company only suggests that it might "help".

First, while the manufacturer's specific "combination" of these nutrients may be creative, it will be found that most, if not all, of the same nutrients are present in most other baby formulas. Second, few clinical studies support any suggestion that such a "unique" combination provides any specific health benefit to a baby relative to the use of other baby formulas.

There are few exceptions to this approach to inferred promises of "improved immunity". One that comes to mind is a study carried out in Spain in which babies who were fed a major international infant formula with good levels of long-chain polyunsaturated essential fatty acids (in line with average breast milk levels) were found to experience significantly fewer respiratory illnesses during infancy than infants who were fed formulas with much lower or no content of those particular fatty acids.

Manufacturers' claims that their baby formulas are "unique" are not confined to immune function. This is why a mother must carefully consider what a particular baby formula offers her baby. Asking your family doctor is not always the best solution. Nutrition is not a major part of medical training, and progressive knowledge regarding nutrition continues at a pace that may be difficult for a general practitioner to keep up with. If you ask your family doctor whether he or she considers a particular baby formula to be suitable, he or she will most likely say, "yes," as the doctor probably considers that all baby formulas are more or less the same. Asking for a recommendation rarely achieves the desired result, as the doctor may not wish to be viewed as being partial towards any particular brand of baby formula.

There are five important sections of a baby formula label.

1. The "Ingredients" list. This tells you what is in the formula. Most labels list the ingredients in descending order according to the amount of each ingredient. The first-mentioned ingredient is usually the one present in the greatest quantity.
2. The "Nutrients" list. This lays out how much of each nutrient is provided by the total "ingredients" listed on the label. Often the way the list is presented in various "units" can make it rather difficult for a mother to compare one baby formula to another. I cover more of this later in the book.
3. The preparation instructions and feeding tables. Meticulous care and attention should be taken to follow the preparation instructions. Once again I cover this in more detail later in the book.
4. The manufacturer or marketer of the baby formula. Is it a renowned and dependable one, well recognized for exceptional quality and ethics?
5. The expiration date. Reputable manufacturers of baby formula "guarantee" that if the formula has been stored at all times under proper conditions, a test of the formula will indicate that each of the nutrient values listed on the label will still be met on that product's expiration date. Some ingredients may lose their potency or presence over time. Reputable manufacturers take this into account by including higher quantities of perishable nutrients at the time of manufacture so that the label claim remains true on the expiration date.

Prebiotics and Probiotics. What are They?

Basically a prebiotic is a non-digestible, starch-like fibre, and a probiotic is a "bug".

By definition a prebiotic is:

"A non-digestible food ingredient that beneficially affects the host by selectively stimulating the growth and/or the activity of a limited number of bacteria in the colon."

The criteria used for classification of a food component as a prebiotic are:

- Resistance to digestion, hydrolysis, and fermentation by colonic microflora (bacteria)
- Selective stimulation of growth of one or a limited number of beneficial bacteria in the fæces.

A more scientific definition of a prebiotic is

"A prebiotic is a selectively fermented ingredient that allows specific changes, both in the composition and/or activity in the gastrointestinal microflora that confers benefits upon host wellbeing and health."

(Gibson & Roberfroid, 2004)

Confused? What this definition says is that prebiotic ingredients are rather selective in that they act as "food" to the "good" bacteria in the gut to help them multiply but do not act as a "food" that would help the "bad" bacteria to proliferate.

Bacteria in the baby's gut? Yes. Before Baby was born, its gut (alimentary tract) was sterile (i.e., it contained no bacteria). The moment Baby was born, the gut was "invaded" by bacteria that multiplied into millions, then billions. Not to worry — most of the species of these bacteria live in harmony with us and provide us many benefits. For example, they help improve digestion, enhance mineral absorption, provide some important vitamins, and improve the immune system in terms of effectiveness and intrinsic strength. Some not-so-nice bacteria are present too, but they are mostly kept under control through competition from other bacteria and special mucus layers that line the alimentary tract.

Interestingly, when babies are born naturally through the birth canal, the species of bacteria in their alimentary tracts mimic those of their mothers. When babies arrive by caesarean section, however, the species of bacteria mimic more closely those in the immediate hospital environment. During the first two to three months following birth, the range and predominance of various bacterial species in the alimentary tracts of exclusively breast-fed babies differ to some extent from the range and predominance of various bacterial species in the alimentary tract of babies who are exclusively formula fed. After a baby reaches about nine weeks of age, however, analyses of bacterial strains in the stools can no longer distinguish whether the baby has been breast-fed or formula fed. Once babies are weaned to semisolid and solid foods, there is no significant difference in bacterial species in the alimentary tract.

A clinical study carried out in Sweden and published in the *Journal of Allergy and Clinical Immunology* in late 2011 suggests that the diversity of alimentary tract bacteria species in babies may be more important than which particular species predominate. Researchers found that babies with a low diversity of bacterial species in the alimentary tract during the first months of life were more likely to experience subsequent allergy development. This tends to fit with the *"hygiene hypothesis"* which states that the low prevalence of allergies among children who grow up on farms and in less affluent countries can be attributed to exposure to a high diversity of bacterial species within the children's environments.

Most of the time, we tend to live in harmony with the bacteria that colonise our alimentary tract. Approximately four hundred-plus species of bacteria are present in the alimentary tract, and they number into trillions of bacterial cells. Less well known is the fact that one-half of the dry weight (or one-third of the wet weight) of our stools is made up of both dead and live bacterial cells.

Studies show that certain bacterial strains appear to confer some benefit to infants, and therefore manufacturers have incorporated some of these strains into certain baby formulas. These strains are known as "probiotics". The definition of a probiotic is :

"A live microbial feed supplement that is beneficial to health."

(ESPGHAN Committee on Nutrition, 2004)

Note the mention of the word "live." Therein lies the problem of incorporating beneficial bacterial strains within a baby formula. The specified bacteria must remain live throughout the life of the formula, from manufacture to expiration date in average storage conditions. The bacteria must then pass through the acid medium of the stomach and remain live when they reach the large intestine. As they rarely "colonise" themselves amongst the hundreds of other bacteria within the alimentary tract, they usually must be administered daily in each feeding of the baby formula.

Some studies support manufacturer claims that specific bacterial strains can help babies achieve "better digestive health" and "help improve immunity" Determining how significant are those benefits will require more widespread studies. Other studies suggest that the stool patterns of infants who are fed baby formula that contain probiotics more resemble those of breast-fed babies.

Just keep in mind that for probiotics to exert their beneficial effects, the bacteria must remain alive and active after formula manufacture, retention within the baby formula, passage through the digestive tract, and their eventual arrival within the colon (large intestine). US authorities are drafting new ingredient quality standards for probiotics. These include testing to confirm probiotic identity, purity, and microbe count in order to ensure safety as well as the authenticity of health claims.

Those "Essential" Omega Fatty Acids

"Fatty acids" are the individual molecules that make up the general fats in our diet or are incorporated within many important functions within our bodies. Many of these fatty acids can be manufactured from scratch by metabolic processes within our bodies then further modified to larger fatty acid molecules. Specific enzyme systems within our bodies assist in these modifications. There are some larger fatty acid molecules, however, that are extremely important to our health and wellbeing, yet our bodies lack the enzyme systems to form them. These enzymes must instead be taken in as a part of our diet, and therefore they are known as *"essential fatty acids"* —that is, it is *essential* that they are present within our diet, because our bodies simply are unable to form them.

Although they share the same metabolic enzyme systems, these essential fatty acids are categorized into two groups —the "Omega-6 fatty acids" and the "Omega-3 fatty acids", according to their molecular structure. Both groups are polyunsaturated fatty acids (PUFAs). Those that are present in plant sources (vegetable oils) are the Omega-6 linoleic acid (LA) and the Omega-3 alpha-linolenic acid (aLA). In theory the enzyme systems in our bodies are able to metabolize these PUFAs through the addition of more carbon atoms and greater "desaturation" to form larger molecules known as "long-chain polyunsaturated fatty acids" (LCPUFAs). The body's ability to have them undergo this metabolism is very restricted; therefore these LCPUFAs also must be present in our diet.

The key Omega-6 LCPUFA is arachidonic acid (ARA). The key Omega-3 LCPUFAs are eicosapentaenoic acid (EPA) and docosahexaenoic acid (DHA).

A baby's brain weighs about 350 g at birth but rapidly increases in size over the next twelve months to weigh approximately 1000 g. A slower rate of brain growth continues to take place during the second year of life, and the weight of the brain is approximately 1200 g when a baby reaches two years of age. Not much brain growth occurs after that, as the average adult male brain weighs approximately 1400 g and the adult female brain weighs approximately 1250 g. My wife explains to me that women use their brains more efficiently!

From the end of the second trimester of pregnancy (at about six months of pregnancy), the developing baby's brain begins to incorporate increasing amounts of Omega-3 DHA and Omega-6 ARA LCPUFAs, and this rapid uptake of these two essential fatty acids continues until two years of age before slowing in the third year of life. Note: The brain does not take in the PUFAs linoleic acid and alpha-linolenic acid.

In 1986 research was published that provided evidence that Omega-3 fatty acids were essential for brain and eye development. In the US the 1990s were designated *"The Decade of the Brain"*, by President G H W Bush and substantial government funding was made available to researchers. The aim may have been to better understand the human brain as a means to improve computers, but the research performed was very valuable in developing an understanding of the benefits to babies that accrue from their receiving an adequate intake of LCPUFA essential fatty acids.

In 2000 clinical studies began to be published in key, peer-reviewed medical journals revealing the significant benefits in mental development index (MDI) scores in babies who were fed baby formula that contained adequate amounts of the LCPUFAs Omega-3 DHA and Omega-6 ARA. MDI scoring is similar to IQ scoring, and the average score is 100. Babies who had been fed formula with LCPUFA during their first seventeen weeks achieved, on average, at eighteen months of age MDI scores seven points higher than babies fed the same formula without the LCPUFA content (the "control" formula). The fact that 26 percent of these babies scored 115 (seventeen points higher than the average for the babies on the control formula) prompted *Scientific American* magazine to take the unprecedented step of highlighting the study as a *"Formula for Intelligence?"* The researchers commented: "These data support a long-term cognitive advantage of infant DHA supply during the first 4 months of life."

High intelligence scores were not the only benefit gained by babies who received high adequate amounts of DHA. Studies published that same year showed that babies who were fed formula that contained LCPUFA had significantly better visual function at twelve months of age than babies on the control formula (without DHA+ARA). The following year (2001), the *Journal of Pediatrics* published a clinical study that found a significant connection between DHA in a baby's diet and language performance and perception at nine months of age.

Grants from the National Institutes of Health in the US supported these studies, and further studies conducted at the Retina Foundation of the Southwest, in Dallas, Texas, confirmed greater visual and neural development in babies who were fed formula that contained DHA. The longer (up to twelve months of age) babies were fed formula with adequate levels of DHA, the more their visual skills developed.

Adequacy of LCPUFA in a Baby's Diet

I keep mentioning "adequate" intake. In the National Institutes of Health-supported studies, the researchers based both the DHA and the ARA levels in the baby formula at the median levels of pooled breast milk from various countries. As Mead Johnson Nutrition earlier had been awarded a patent for a special blend of vegetable oils that provided a fatty acid profile very similar to that in breast milk, the researchers at the Retina Foundation of the Southwest approached Mead Johnson Nutrition to provide the baby formula Enfamil® as the control formula for their studies. Their choice was probably further influenced by an earlier study in Canada that showed that this baby formula with its new vegetable oil blend also had been shown to provide babies with eye development closer to that of breast-fed babies than had been achieved with earlier baby formulas.

The researchers also requested that Mead Johnson Nutrition produce for their studies batches of the control formula with added DHA at a level of 17 mg/100 kcal and ARA at a level of 34 mg/100 kcal. These levels were based on average levels of DHA and ARA found in pooled samples of breast milk in Texas and various other locations around the world. These levels also approximated recommendations by the Food and Agriculture Organization of the United Nations (FAO) and the World Health Organization regarding the incorporation of LCPUFAs into baby formula.

The results of their studies probably represent the most significant advancement in the knowledge of the impact that nutrient intake can have on eye and brain development during babyhood. These studies were certainly recognized as reinforcing the need for "Evidence-based Nutrition", which is akin to "Evidence-based Medicine" wherein acceptance of effectiveness requires well-controlled, randomized clinical studies that are able to give reproducible results.

Previously, long-term studies had demonstrated that inadequate intake of iron during critical periods of brain development in babies adversely affected scholastic achievement many years later, despite vigorous iron therapy in early childhood. In fact a further follow-up with this group showed that at adolescence these children still had low scholastic achievement relative to their peers who had not experienced insufficient iron intake during babyhood.

In studies carried out in the late 1990s and published in peer-reviewed medical journals in subsequent years, researchers at the Retina Foundation of the Southwest demonstrated that adequate dietary intake of the LCPUFAs DHA and ARA during the first twelve months of life could result in significantly enhanced eye and brain development. In multicentre studies performed by other researchers in the more western states of the US with Similac® (Abbott) as the control baby formula, to which was added only 9 mg/100 kcal of DHA and 25 mg/100 kcal of ARA, no measurable differences were observed between babies on the tested formula relative to the control formula. This was probably the first signal that there has to be an "adequate" amount of LCPUFA dietary intake for a baby to show any noticeable benefit. Remember that the studies carried out at the Retina Foundation of the Southwest were based on higher levels of LCPUFAs — DHA at a level of 17 mg/100 kcal and ARA at a level of 34 mg/100 kcal.

It remains a mystery as to why Abbott went on to incorporate, globally, only the low level of DHA and ARA into their marketed baby formulas, when researchers in the western states of the US already had shown no measurable benefit for the babies who would consume those formulas. Their baby-formula levels of DHA and ARA also fall well below recommendations outlined by the FAO/WHO in their 1994 publication "Fats and Oils in Human Nutrition: Report of a Joint Expert Consultation". It becomes confusing when the same manufacturer took out full newspaper advertisements in Singapore in 2001 claiming: *"Study published in Pediatrics shows NO BENEFIT in adding AA & DHA to term infant formula."* The study was their own (mentioned above), using formula with only 9 mg/100 kcal of DHA and 25 mg/100 kcal of ARA added. Soon afterward, however, Abbott began to add the LCPUFAs into their baby formulas globally albeit at the low levels of 10 mg DHA/100 kcal and 21 mg ARA/100 kcal.

"The eyes are the window to the brain"

In the article "Impact of Early Dietary Intake and Blood Composition of Long-Chain Polyunsaturated Fatty Acids on Later Visual Development," published in the prestigious *Journal of Pediatric Gastroenterology and Nutrition* in 2000, a group of internationally renowned researchers explained: *"Because the central nervous system including the retina is derived embryologically from neuroectoderm, assessment of visual development in early childhood directly reflects development progression in the brain."*

The retina's response to light travels from the eyes to the primary visual cortex, which is situated at the very rear of the brain. Any response to changing patterns during testing requires brain signals to travel through to the front of the brain for "assessment" and then to the eyes to have them move in relation to the stimulus. This is how the measurement of visual acuity development also reflects more general brain development.

As a baby's response to visual stimuli now can be accurately measured with more advanced techniques, such tests represent an important non-invasive method of establishing the degree of brain development during babyhood.

Using the more sophisticated testing methods to measure the degree of visual development, researchers at the Retina Foundation of the Southwest have clearly established from various periods of feeding baby formula with DHA and ARA during babyhood the following:

1. The feeding of baby formula with DHA and ARA at adequate levels results in significantly more advanced visual development compared to the feeding of baby formula that does not contain LCPUFAs.

2. The length of time during babyhood that a baby receives adequate levels of LCPUFAs is directly related to the degree of eye development (and hence brain development) in that baby.

In recognition of this research, which formed the basis of evidence-based nutrition, the European Food Safety Authority (EFSA) on January 22, 2009 gave its Summary of Opinion regarding permissible claims for the role of DHA in visual development of infants. The EFSA categorically stated,

> *"In order to bear the claim (DHA contributes to the visual development of infants) a formula should contain at least 0.3% of the total fatty acids as decosahexaenoic acid."*

Unfortunately, despite the weight of evidence, very few baby formula manufacturers globally provide this level of LCPUFAs in their formulas. Perhaps it is a question of cost, as the addition of LCPUFAs to a baby formula adds a very significant increase in the cost of the materials. It may be rather tempting for manufacturers to include less than adequate levels of LCPUFAs in a baby formula, simply to be able to say that they include some.

Globally, Mead Johnson Nutrition is consistent in ensuring their Enfamil® baby formulas contain adequate levels of LCPUFAs. This is not the case with all manufacturers. For example, in the US, Nestlé markets their baby formula with levels of LCPUFAs almost identical to those in Mead Johnson Nutrition's Enfamil® LIPIL, and for many years the Nestlé home page stated,

> *"The levels of DHA & ARA in Good Start Supreme DHA & ARA are recommended by experts and are similar to levels that have been shown in studies to support brain and eye development."*
> *"These levels are also comparable to the levels specified by the World Health Organization (WHO)."*

Throughout Asia and in Europe, however, Nestlé marketed their Nan® 1 baby formula with the low LCPUFA levels of only 11.7 mg DHA/100 kcal and 11.7 mg ARA/100 kcal. The rather low amount of ARA is interesting, as it represents only 0.22 percent of the total fatty acids in the formula. In 2007 the

American Society for Nutrition published in their journal, the *American Journal of Clinical Nutrition*, a meta-analysis of sixty-five studies from numerous countries around the world that involved 2,474 women and analysed the mean (average) breast milk concentrations of DHA and ARA in each study. Not one of those sixty-five studies had a mean ARA level below 0.24 percent of total fatty acids. The range of mean ARA levels was from 0.24 percent to 1 percent of total fatty acids.

      <u>Footnote:</u> Unfortunately for mothers in Australia and New Zealand, Mead Johnson Nutrition does not market their baby formulas in those countries. No well baby formulas sold in either Australia or New Zealand contain what would be regarded as "adequate" levels of DHA. For my granddaughters (in Australia), the contents of one capsule of "Fish Oil 1000" were squeezed into each litre of prepared baby formula.

How Can I Tell How Much DHA a Baby Formula Contains?

Variations on how manufacturers express their nutrients content can confuse mothers. A nutrients chart usually features in the left-most column a statement of the food energy provided by the formula, followed by a list of nutrients, starting with protein content, fat content, and carbohydrate (mainly starches and sugars) content, and then a long list of specific nutrients, including numerous vitamins and minerals.

Energy provision is expressed in either kilocalories (kcal) or kilojoules (kj). The conversion factor is 1 kcal = 4.18 kj. In other words if a specific amount of baby formula provides 120 kcal, this is the equivalent of 502 kj (120 x 4.18 = 502). If a company claims a specific amount of a baby formula provides 600 kj, this is the equivalent of 144 kcal (600 ÷ 4.18 = 144).

Following the name of each nutrient (or sometimes in a separate column) the label states the units of weight measurement that the numerical values in the following columns claim for each individual nutrient.

- g (grams) = 1,000 milligrams or one million micrograms
- mg (milligrams) = 1,000 micrograms
- mcg (micrograms)

Often vitamins such as vitamin D or vitamin E are expressed in "iu".
- iu (international units)

The following columns list the amount (by weight) of each nutrient in the amount of baby formula stated at the head of each column.

- Per 100 g   (of powder)
- Per 100 ml   (of prepared formula)
- Per 1 litre, or per 1,000 ml (of prepared formula)
- Per 100 kcal   (of energy)

This is where it can start to become difficult to compare baby formula nutrient details from can label information. Sometimes a formula may have less fat content (some even lower than the fat content of breast milk), and the manufacturer will use a slightly bigger scoop to ensure that Baby receives an appropriate level of daily energy intake. Lower fat baby formulas use more powder per prepared bottle, and therefore you get through your can of baby formula sooner. This is because each gram of fat provides two-and-one-fourth times more energy than does one gram of protein or one gram of carbohydrate.

This is also why you cannot compare "per 100 g" values from one can's label with "per 100 ml" values on another can's label. As babies drink "energy" according to their needs, it's best to compare labels using "per 100 kcal". Many baby formula labels, however, do not provide this nutrient value listing. What should you do? Look at the energy (kcal) value under "per 100 g." If it is, say, 530 kcal, then to calculate nutrient values per 100 kcal, the conversion factor would be 100 ÷ 530 = 0.19. Multiplying the "per 100 g" value for a particular nutrient by 0.19 will convert the value of that nutrient to per 100 kcal.

Some examples calculated from can labels are:

Similac® Advance Eye Q Plus (Abbott)
DHA: 10.5 mg/100 kcal
ARA: 20.9 mg/100 kcal

Nan® 1 (Nestlé)
DHA: 11.8 mg/100 kcal
ARA: 11.8 mg/100 kcal

Enfamil® A+/Enfamil® LIPIL (Mead Johnson Nutrition)
DHA: 17.0 mg/100 kcal
ARA: 34.0 mg/100 kcal

Note: As some branded baby formulas differ from country to country, it is wise to use the calculations outlined above to establish the relevant nutrient levels in your country.

There is "Omega-3" .... and then there is "Omega-3"

There is a lot of confusion among the general public, and even among some doctors, as to what is referred to as "Omega-3" fatty acids. This occurs usually due to a lack of differentiation between Omega-3 polyunsaturated fatty acid (PUFA) and long-chain polyunsaturated fatty acid (LCPUFA).

Omega-3 PUFA comes from plant-based sources such as flaxseed oil and soy oil. Omega-3 LCPUFA comes from animal-based sources such as fish-oil and from algae. Algal-based sources provide Omega-3 LCPUFA in a form that is suitable for vegetarians.

The human body can metabolize Omega-3 PUFA to Omega-3 LCPUFA. Unfortunately, however, studies over the past two decades clearly have shown that such conversion is of a very low order indeed. Provide in a breast-feeding mother's diet some oily fish, and her breast milk DHA is elevated. Provide in her diet flaxseed oil, and there is no increase whatsoever in her breast milk DHA. Sophisticated scientific studies indicate that when Omega-3 PUFA is taken in the diet, a very large amount of it is very quickly used as a source of energy for the body.

Studies generally agree that whole-body conversion of α-linolenic acid (Omega-3 PUFA) to DHA is below 5 percent in humans and depends on the concentration of Omega-6 fatty acids and LCPUFAs in the diet. High amounts of Omega-6 fatty acids (for example, linoleic acid, which is prevalent in most vegetable oils) in the diet tend to further reduce the conversion rate of Omega-3 PUFA to Omega-3 LCPUFA.

Twenty-five percent of dietary α-linolenic acid Omega-3 PUFA is completely oxidized within the body (to provide energy) within the first twenty-four hours and reaches 60 percent by seven days. Much of the remaining α-linolenic acid serves as a source of acetate for synthesis of saturates and monounsaturates, with very little stored as α-linolenic acid.

During the last trimester of pregnancy and the first twelve months of a baby's life, there is a large accumulation of the Omega-3 LCPUFA DHA (docosahexaenoic acid) in a baby's brain, but there is no such accumulation of other Omega-3 LCPUFAs, such as EPA (eicosapentaenoic acid), nor is there any presence in the brain of Omega-3 PUFA (α-linolenic acid). This emphasizes the need for "adequacy" of DHA in a baby's diet throughout babyhood.

Choline

Choline is a vitamin-like compound, and the need for such compounds increases during periods of rapid tissue growth, such as in the doubling of body weight during the first year of babyhood.

Choline is the precursor of major components of all body cells, including the neurons and the glial cells of the brain; therefore an adequate supply of choline is crucial during the development of the nervous system. Choline is also necessary for the formation of acetylcholine, an important neurotransmitter within the brain and nervous system.

A choline-based compound, phosphatidylcholine, is the predominant (greater than 50 percent) phospholipid in most mammalian membranes. The rapidly growing baby's brain therefore has a high requirement for choline for the formation of phosphatidylcholine for incorporation into new membranes.

Mammalian studies have shown that choline supports the development of long-term memory and that such development during the period of babyhood has a long-term beneficial effect through to adulthood.

Breast milk contains high levels of choline. Concentrations of choline in the serum (of the blood) are more than threefold to sevenfold in newborns than they are in adults. Prior to the mid-1990s, analytical methods were not able to measure the choline level in all components of breast milk. In 1988, following the reassessment of the choline content of breast milk, the Food and Nutrition Board of the Institute of Medicine in the US concluded that the average total choline content of breast milk to be higher, at 160 ml per litre. They used this new level to establish the "Adequate Intake" levels for babies. This equates to 24 mg per 100 kcal.

Many quality baby formulas increased their choline levels to reflect this new appreciation of the higher choline levels found in breast milk. Unfortunately many baby formulas still have not yet done so. It therefore is wise to check the nutrient tables on baby formula labels to determine whether a particular baby formula contains an adequate intake level of choline.

Once again if the nutrient table on the label does not have a listing expressed in "per kcal" (remember that babies drink energy/calories), then use the usual conversion from the value in the "per 100 g" column.

Look at the energy (kcal) value under "per 100 g." If it is, say, 530 kcal, then to calculate nutrient values per 100 kcal, the conversion factor would be 100 ÷ 530 = 0.19. Multiplying the per 100 g value for a particular nutrient by 0.19 will convert the value of that nutrient to per 100 kcal.

Some examples calculated from can labels are:

Similac® Advance Eye Q Plus (Abbott)
Choline: 15 mg/100 kcal

Nan® 1 (Nestlé)
Choline: 18 mg/100 kcal

Enfamil A®+ / Enfamil® LIPIL (Mead Johnson Nutrition)
Choline: 24 mg/100 kcal

Note: As some branded baby formulas differ from country-to-country, it is wise to use the calculations outlined above to establish the relevant nutrient levels in your country.

IRON — Ensuring Baby has Enough

The long-term consequences of iron deficiency during babyhood make it so important for babies to receive an adequate intake of iron. It also is important that a baby maintains a good iron status at all times throughout the duration of babyhood.

> *"Brain growth is time dependent. Different developmental processes occur at specific chronological ages, and once the time for a phase of growth has passed, it cannot be restarted."*
>
> **Morgan (1990)**

Iron is an essential cofactor for numerous proteins involved in neuronal function. Iron deficiency anæmia is associated with neurological disturbances. Iron deficiency causes lower cognitive, motor, attention, and developmental scores, including failure to respond to test stimuli, short attention span, unhappiness, increased fearfulness, withdrawal, and increased body tension.

More than twenty-five years ago, it had become established that insufficiency of iron during babyhood resulted in neurodevelopment delays that could not be reversed with later iron therapy. The adverse effects of iron deficiency on baby development are well documented. Decreased growth rate, lower mental and motor test scores, increased susceptibility to infection, behavioural abnormalities, and decreased scholastic achievement in later childhood are all manifestations of insufficient iron intake during the first twelve months of life.

As long as a mother has a good iron status, her baby is born with iron stores beyond its body's immediate requirements. A baby who weighs 3.5 kg at birth has a total of about 250 mg of total body iron. Of this, 175 mg of iron is in the hæmoglobin of the red blood cells; 15 mg is in myoglobin and enzymes; and there is about 60 mg in iron stores within the body. Up until four months of age, there is little change in the level of total body iron, but the distribution changes. There is now more iron in the red blood cells as the baby has grown, but it has reduced significantly the iron stores in the body.

At about four months of age, a baby has a far greater need for iron as the baby continues his or her rapid rate of growth to reach about 10 kg of body weight by one year of age. After about four months of age, a progressive shift occurs from an abundance of iron to the marginal iron reserves that characterize the period of continued rapid growth. This transition from feast to famine is regarded as the "window of vulnerability" to iron deficiency. This is why formula-fed babies require iron-fortified baby formulas.

Some manufacturers of baby formulas believe that a good level of iron fortification is not required during the first few months of a baby's life and therefore do not further increase iron levels in their formulas until Stage 2 (follow-on) formulas. Others believe that maintaining good iron fortification throughout the entire period of babyhood can help avoid body iron stores from becoming too marginal. This certainly makes sense in Asian countries, where iron deficiency is endemic. Clinical studies have demonstrated that good levels of iron intake from baby formula throughout the whole of babyhood, right from birth, are well tolerated by babies.

Once again, if the nutrient table on the formula label does not have a listing expressed in "per kcal" (remember that babies drink energy/calories), then use the usual conversion from the value in the "per 100 g" column.

Look at the energy (kcal) value under "per 100 g." If it is, say, 530 kcal, then to calculate nutrient values per 100 kcal, the conversion factor would be $100 \div 530 = 0.19$. Multiplying the per 100 g value for a particular nutrient by 0.19 will convert the value of that nutrient to per 100 kcal.

Some calculated examples of iron content from Stage 1 formula can labels are:

Similac® Advance Eye Q Plus (Abbott)
Iron: 1.23 mg/100 kcal

Nan® 1 (Nestlé)
Iron: 1.00 mg/100 kcal

Enfamil® A+ / Enfamil® LIPIL (Mead Johnson Nutrition)
Iron: 1.23 mg/100 kcal

Note: As some branded baby formulas differ from country-to-country, it is wise to use the calculations outlined above to establish the relevant nutrient levels in your country.

How Accurately do I Need to Prepare a Baby Formula?

Baby formula manufacturers set out clear instructions on the labels of their formula powder cans for preparation of the product for feeding to your baby. For feeding during the first six months of life, it is very important to follow these instructions exactly. The manufacturer has designed the size of the accompanying scoop to accurately measure just how much powder you should mix with the stipulated volume of previously boiled, then cooled, water, and the guide will ensure that your baby has the necessary water balance.

Each scoopful of powder should be a level scoopful. When the scoop is filled, wipe a clean table knife across the mouth of the scoop to return any surplus powder to the can. Failure to do this leaves heaped scoopfuls, and therefore more solids (powder) are added to the stipulated amount of water, which forms a stronger mixture than the manufacturer intends for your baby. Over a period of time, there is a possibility that this could result in a water deficit in your baby, which will force the kidneys to work harder.

When taking scoopfuls of powder from the can, do not hard-press the filled scoop against the inside of the can. Once again, the scoop volume is calculated for loose powder, and if powder is crammed or hard-packed into the scoop, your baby will receive a stronger mixture of prepared formula than intended.

When preparing formula and using the recommended number of scoopfuls of powder with the appropriate amount of previously boiled, then cooled, water do not be tempted to add another scoopful of powder "for luck" or for the intention of giving Baby an extra growth boost. Adding extra scoopfuls of powder over and above the number stipulated in the mixing instructions quickly can create a water deficit in your baby. Similarly, some mothers can get a little competitive when comparing their baby's growth to the babies of friends and acquaintances and feel they can gain a competitive advantage by adding an extra scoopful of powder when preparing their own baby's formula. Such actions, however, can result in adverse health reactions in babies.

Bluntly, never deviate from the preparation instructions on the formula label. In hot climates or when Baby may have a feverish condition, more water may be required, but you should always provide this separately from prepared formula by giving your baby previously boiled, then cooled, water alone. Do *not* use fruit juices.

Why it can be Difficult to Compare Breast Milk with Baby Formula

Authorities in most countries, guided by the WHO Code of Marketing, clearly prohibit baby formula manufacturers or marketers from making any claims for their products relative to breast milk. That makes a whole lot of sense for a number of reasons, not the least being that a baby formula is standardised for all cans of that specific formula under the same branded label produced by a manufacturer, whereas breast milk is anything but standardized. Components of breast milk vary over time, from soon after birth through six months, one year, or two years after the start of lactation. A mother's diet can influence some components of breast milk, and composition of breast milk varies from early in each feeding to late in each feeding. Furthermore, as outlined earlier, breast feeding can be limited to 750 ml to 850 ml per day for most mothers, whereas a baby older than three months may consume one litre of baby formula per day.

Nevertheless, this does not seem to daunt the release by breast-feeding advocates of "studies" that tend to show that individuals who were breast-fed as babies were superior to those who were fed baby formula. Such "studies," however, rarely give consideration to any or all of the following:

- As it can take about three years to collate all the data, submit it to a journal for publication, and eventually have it published, then for a study on, for example, outcomes of scholastic achievement measured during adolescence, a period of about eighteen years has elapsed between the feeding that youth received as a baby and the publication date of the study.
- Following breast-feeding or formula feeding, each individual has had varied feeding patterns and daily nutrient intake.

- Over the intervening eighteen years or so, the dietary habits and food choices of breast-feeding mothers could have changed considerably according to specific warnings and recommendations, such as *"Avoid fish, it might have mercury in it"; "Avoid saturated fats and use vegetable oils"; "Avoid eggs, as they may increase your cholesterol levels";* and so on. Many of these exhortations might have been largely misguided, but they nevertheless may have changed the mothers' eating habits, as the plethora of new fast food outlets also may have.

- Over the intervening eighteen years or so, baby formulas have progressed rapidly in their sophistication of important nutrients, so that baby formulas in studies commenced long ago have no real relevancy to today's quality baby formulas. This is a good reason to check the dates in the study of when the baby formula was fed. If it was a shorter term study, over how many years ago was it conducted? After all, important Omega-3 LCPUFAs were not included in commercial baby formulas until the year 2000.

Formulas for Premature and LBW Babies

A baby is considered "premature" when he or she is born before the end of the thirty-seventh week of gestation. A low birth-weight (LBW) baby is one who weighs less than 2,500 g (2.5 kg) at birth. There is phenomenal growth in the foetus during the last few weeks of pregnancy. Therefore a baby born prematurely has not experienced the significant growth or the maturity from which a full-term baby has benefited.

Interestingly, when a mother gives birth to her baby prematurely, her breast milk contains a significantly higher amount of protein than the breast milk of a mother who gives birth to a full-term baby. This is also true of many other nutrients, including calcium, zinc, copper, sodium, and chlorine. There also appears to be significant host-defence benefits from feeding premature babies their own mothers' breast milk.

Recent advances in medicine, nutrition, and controlled environment have enabled neonatologists to maintain life in babies born very prematurely. Very low birth-weight (VLBW) and extremely low birth-weight (ELBW) infants require fortification of breast milk with multi-nutrient supplementation or the addition of specialized (purpose-formulated) premature baby formula.

Low birth-weight (LBW) babies weigh less than 2500 g (five pounds, eight ounces), regardless of the length of gestation. Very low birth-weight (VLBW) babies weigh less than 1500 g at birth, and extremely low birth-weight (ELBW) babies weigh less than 1000 g at birth. Many mothers of ELBW or VLBW babies have insufficient breast milk to fulfill their baby's needs. For this reason quality purpose-formulated preterm baby formulas play an important role.

The low birth-weight baby has unique nutritional needs, including:

• Higher protein needs
• Increased energy requirements

- A need for utilisable carbohydrates
- A need for easily digestible fat
- Greater calcium needs
- A need for low osmolar load
- A need for specific levels of vitamins/minerals

Regular "well infant" formulas cannot adequately meet these special needs.

Premature babies have the following special nutritional requirements that regular starter infant formulas cannot meet:

- Increased caloric density (due to very small stomach size)
- Increased protein intake for rapid growth
- Avoidance of hyperosmolar feeds
- Reduced lactose loading (too much lactose may cause osmotic diarrhœa)
- A readily assimilable fat source
- Low iron intake
- Increased calcium and phosphorus levels for bone growth
- Increased sodium intake
- Increased vitamin E

Nothing can be done to make a regular starter (Stage 1) infant formula well suited to the nutritional and feeding requirements of premature and VLBW babies. Any attempt to modify a regular starter formula to meet one parameter usually worsens one or more other elements relative to required parameters. For this reason a baby formula for the feeding of preterm and VLBW babies must be "purpose-formulated" in order to meet the established nutritional and feeding requirements for these babies.

Babies born before thirty-two to thirty-four weeks of gestation (usually VLBW) lack coordination of sucking, swallowing, and breathing, and therefore are usually fed by nasogastric (via a tube inserted through the nose to the stomach) or orogastric (via a tube through the mouth to the stomach) gavage feeding, which uses a large syringe inserted into the end of the gavage tube.

Preterm babies who are born with a weight less than 1,000 g (ELBW) or who are critically ill require parenteral (intravenous) feeding as their main source of nutrition.

Obviously then, VLBL and ELBL babies are under the supervision of a neonatologist and the constant care of neonatal specialist staff within the neonatal intensive care unit of the hospital until they have attained satisfactory growth and development milestones.

Earlier, premature, LBW and VLBW babies tended to continue to lag behind the growth and development milestones of full-term babies, even when adjusted to PMA (post-menstrual age or age since conception). Then in 2005 the *Journal of Pediatrics* published the findings of a double-blind clinical study that involved 245 VLBW infants, which demonstrated that babies who received premature baby formula that contained LCPUFAs (once again, at "adequate" levels) achieved much improved growth and development:

"The more important finding is that the addition of these levels of DHA and ARA to the diets of preterm infants improved their mental and psychomotor development at eighteen months after term, compared to preterm infants fed unsupplemented formula."

"These results are of considerable importance because very and extremely low birth weight preterm infants remain at risk for subnormal weight and height through childhood and perhaps into adulthood."

Clandinin, Diersen-Schade, et al. J Pediatrics, 2005; 146:461-468

This finding reinforces, yet again, the importance of babies receiving a baby formula that contains "adequate" amounts of the LCPUFAs DHA & ARA.

The Frequently Crying Baby

As every parent knows, babies tend to cry a lot during their first three to four months of life. If the crying is particularly persistent, and especially if it is associated with gastro-oesophageal reflux (GOR or GER), it wise to discuss this with your pædiatrician or your general practitioner. "*Gastro-oesophageal reflux*" is a backward or return flow of the contents of the stomach and duodenal into the oesophagus. Only when the reflux of stomach contents reaches the mouth is this referred to as "*regurgitation*". Regurgitation is the sudden and effortless return of small amounts of undigested stomach or oesophageal contents into the pharynx or the mouth. These contents commonly spill out of the mouth (often referred to as "spillage" or "spitting up"). It is estimated that up to 50 percent of babies younger than three months of age have frequent mild vomiting due to reflux. For most babies this is not a problem, although it can cause significant parental anxiety and stress.

Some babies are not distressed or affected by their reflux. With adequate parental reassurance and support, many babies cope and outgrow this problem. Regarded as "*physiological reflux*", this is a normal condition and generally resolves itself in about 99 percent of cases by twelve months of age.

Reflux only becomes a problem when the baby displays signs of associated complications. When complications develop, the condition is referred to as "*clinical reflux*" or "*pathological reflux*". Complications may include "failure to thrive", oesophagitis (inflammation of the oesophagus), and respiratory problems such as apnœa (temporary cessation of breathing), wheezing, and aspiration (inhalation of the reflux material).

Only a small percentage of babies suffer complications. Significant gastro-oesophageal reflux disease (GORD) occurs only in one in five hundred infants but tends to be over-diagnosed.

The newborn baby has to deal with four main issues. The oesophagus, through which food travels from the mouth to the stomach, is very short, which makes it easier for refluxed material to reach the mouth. This distance increases as the infant grows. Very young infants have small stomachs, and rapid or high-volume feeding can fill the stomach quickly, which increases gastric pressure. Lack of muscle strength or inadequate nervous system development can cause the sphincter muscle, which separates the oesophagus and stomach, to relax transiently and allow stomach contents to flow back up the oesophagus and into the mouth. The basal pressure of this sphincter muscle increases to adult levels by two to three months of age. *"Peristalsis"* is the term for the progressive muscular contractions of the oesophagus that actively transport food to the stomach. The immaturity of newborn babies, however, through motor abnormalities and incomplete peristaltic waves, can contribute to an inability of normal peristalsis to remove material from the oesophagus.

Excessive crying in a newborn is more likely to be a developmental adjustment period due to an inability to produce enough lactase (the enzyme that digests lactose, the sugar in milk) to cope with the volume of lactose the newborn receives from either breast milk or baby formula. This is surprisingly common in the first three to four months of a baby's life. The molecular structure of lactose is too large to be able to be transported (absorbed) through the wall of the small intestine, and its molecules must first be broken down (digested) by the specific enzyme lactose to produce two smaller molecules, glucose and galactose, which then can be transported through the wall of the small intestine to the blood vessels that take them to the liver. If insufficient lactase is present, some of the lactose from the feed passes through the small intestine unchanged and enters the large intestine. As pointed out in the section on probiotics, billions of bacteria reside in the large intestine, and they find this undigested lactose a wonderful energy source, which they then release by the fermentation of the lactose. In the process the bacteria also release what are referred to as "short-chain fatty acids" (although they are not really "fats"), which are absorbed from the large intestine and provide another source of energy for the baby.

In this way not all of the energy value of the lactose that the baby could not digest is lost, but this fermentation process produces the gases carbon dioxide, hydrogen, and methane. In young babies excessive production of these intestinal gases can give rise to abdominal discomfort due to distension of the large intestine.

The degree of fermentation can be determined by a breath hydrogen test, which only can be performed in a research or teaching hospital environment. Whereas carbon dioxide and methane can be metabolized within the body, hydrogen gas cannot and is excreted in expired air from the lungs after traveling through the bloodstream. The excess hydrogen in the expired air is detected and measured. A hydrogen breath test is an excellent non-invasive technique to measure the degree of lactose maldigestion.

Surprisingly, early in babyhood a large proportion of babies exhibit signs of undigested lactose that reach the large intestine to be fermented by the resident bacteria there. This usually manifests itself in the form of *"colicky behaviour"* during the first three months or so of infancy, and breath hydrogen testing has confirmed this. This usually resolves itself naturally by about four months of age.

The crying episodes of colicky behaviour arise from the intense pain a baby experiences from the distension of the large intestine by the fermentation gases. When a baby is born, pain transmission is already present, but it is not until the baby is about eight months old that the nervous system has fully developed the mechanisms to help suppress pain. Therefore the baby feels this pain more acutely than does an adult, who usually can resolve such discomfort by the passing of flatulence.

"Although pain transmission mechanisms are present at birth, pain inhibitory mechanisms are immature and pain may be experienced at lower levels of stimulation by nerves with lower thresholds."

"Thus during the first 8 months of life, infants lack fully developed pain inhibitory processes."

"The infant also lacks the ability to inhibit behavioural responses to pain — such as crying."

"The most common complaint brought to doctors during the first 3 months of a baby's life is crying …….. infants lack fully developed inhibitory mechanisms, and crying can continue unchecked."

Hamilton, Zeigler. Visceral Pain in Infants.
Journal of Pediatrics. 1994; 125:S95-S102.

The mechanism of a baby's reaction to the fermentation within the large intestine of undigested lactose was understood by Canadian researchers in 1984, but the frequency of its occurrence was not appreciated until the 1988 publication in the *Journal of Pediatrics* of a study by research doctors in Adelaide, Australia. They defined *"colicky behaviour"* as follows:

- Mild colic: unexplained crying or fussiness that was easily ameliorated.
- Moderate colic: episodes of sustained crying in which attempts at comforting were only partially successful.
- Severe colic: prolonged, intense periods of crying or screaming that failed to respond to comfort measures.

In this study of 122 newborn babies, eighty-three (68 percent) of these babies developed symptoms of colicky behaviour. The average age of onset was 2.6 weeks, but the range of onset was from birth up to eight weeks of age. At six weeks of age, 62 percent of the babies were affected, but by three months of age only 34 percent of the babies were still affected. It made no difference whether the baby was breast-fed or formula fed. After all, both provide about the same amount of lactose to the baby.

When you are pacing up and down throughout the night trying to comfort your crying baby, it may be difficult for you to keep reminding yourself that by four months of age this type of crying will no longer be an issue. As Baby continues to grow and the feeding volumes have levelled, Baby will produce enough lactase enzyme to digest all of the lactose sugar of milk that arrives in the small intestine.

It is also those nights after nights spent trying to comfort a crying baby — as well as desperately seeking their own sleep and comfort during that first three to four months — that drives parents to blame their choice of formula as the culprit. Their solution? Try a different Stage 1 starter formula. But the crying persists (after all they all have about the same amount of lactose), which prompts many parents to move to yet another Stage 1 starter formula. Changing baby formulas may persist for most of those first three to four months until Baby settles — which usually occurs when Baby has grown enough to be able digest within the small intestine all of the lactose provided in the formula he or she now receives.

If you feel it may take a change of formula to reduce your baby's crying, you might consider changing to a special baby formula that is either low in lactose or is regarded as "lactose-free". This change should not be taken lightly and should be discussed with your pædiatrician. Just remember that for a formula to have either a low lactose level or to be regarded as lactose-free, the lactose sugar of the milk content has been replaced by other "sugars", usually maltodextrins or glucose polymers. More important, you should take out your trusty calculator again to see whether the specialized baby formula provides adequate levels of LCPUFAs, choline, and iron as well as a whey protein to casein protein ratio of 60:40, which is similar to that in breast milk.

Now it is All up to You

Over my decades of experiences in many countries, I've gained an appreciation that babies around the world are surprisingly similar. What differs greatly
is their immediate environment. Attitudes, accommodation, ready availability
of clean water, and standards of sanitation and hygiene are just some of the
factors that can affect good baby-feeding practices.

I have attempted to provide you with a reasonably comprehensive
understanding of what you should consider when choosing a baby formula.
Please remember that this book relates only to well babies who have no un-
derlying health problems, congenital defects, or special nutritional needs. In no
way does it constitute an alternative to the sage advice of your family doctor
or pædiatrician when you have concern or reason to feel a need for his or her
assistance.

The purchase of a baby formula is only a first step. In most countries
baby formula comes in powder form. You then must prepare it in the appropriate liquid form to be poured into a nurser (bottle) for feeding to your baby. I
already have emphasized the importance of explicitly following the reconstitu-
tion directions on the can label to help avoid water deficits in your baby. For the
ultimate care of your baby, you also must exercise strict sanitation and hygiene
practices, both with the utensils you use and with the handling of the prepared
formula. A clean water source is important, and the water used for reconstitu-
tion should first be boiled for five minutes, then cooled, before the addition of
the formula powder.

Much of the material I have provided represents information based on
published clinical studies in several areas of nutritional impact on baby development during the period of babyhood. The original "science speak" can be
rather daunting, so I have tried to simplify the terminology as much as possible
without losing the general understanding. I am hopeful that your understanding has been enhanced enough to make educated choices regarding baby

formula selection. As pointed out early in this book, quality baby formulas have become much more sophisticated over the past decade, and these developments are likely to continue. The preceding pages represent "as of 2012" considerations of these developments.

Of course, there are lower-priced baby formulas in the marketplace that maintain their prices by not adding the refinements of nutritional knowledge that have become available over the past decade or so. As in many avenues in life, you usually "get what you pay for" and the information in this book assists you in evaluating that. At the end of the day, however, there is only one start to Life, and that start should be the very best you can provide for your baby. I hope that in some small way I have helped you achieve that.

"It is not just how much you know,
but how much you understand that matters."

www.ingramcontent.com/pod-product-compliance
Lightning Source LLC
Chambersburg PA
CBHW071632170526
45166CB00003B/1294